DIETS TO HELP HYPERTENSION

Hypertension is the medical term for high blood-pressure and can often be directly related to inadequate diet. When hypertension occurs it is a warning sign that must be heeded, and this book explains the simple but effective dietary means that can reduce high blood-pressure and prevent the onset of degenerative cardiovascular disease.

By the same author
NATURE CURE FOR BRONCHITIS AND EMPHYSEMA
NATURE CURE FOR CYSTITIS
NATURE CURE FOR SINUSITIS
THE REALFOOD COOKBOOK (with Vivien Quick)

Also in this series
DIETS TO HELP ACNE *Alan Moyle*
DIETS TO HELP ARTHRITIS *Helen MacFarlane*
DIETS TO HELP BRONCHIAL TROUBLES *Alan Moyle*
DIETS TO HELP CATARRH *Alan Moyle*
DIETS TO HELP COELIACS *Rita Greer*
DIETS TO HELP COLITIS *Joan Lay*
DIETS TO HELP CONTROL CHOLESTEROL *Roger Newman Turner*
DIETS TO HELP CYSTITIS *Ralph McCutcheon*
DIETS TO HELP DIABETICS *Martin Budd*
DIETS TO HELP GALL BLADDER TROUBLES *Nalda Gosling*
DIETS TO HELP HAY FEVER AND ASTHMA *Roger Newman Turner*
DIETS TO HELP HEADACHES *Michael Nightingale*
DIETS TO HELP HEART DISORDERS *Roger Newman Turner*
DIETS TO HELP HYPERTENSION *Clifford Quick*
DIETS TO HELP KIDNEY DISORDERS *Harry Clements*
DIETS TO HELP MULTIPLE SCLEROSIS *Rita Greer*
DIETS TO HELP PSORIASIS *Harry Clements*

DIETS TO HELP
HYPERTENSION

by

CLIFFORD QUICK
M.Sc., D.O., N.D.

THORSONS PUBLISHERS LIMITED
Wellingborough, Northamptonshire

First published 1978
Second Impression 1980
Third Impression 1983
Fourth Impression 1986

ISBN 0 7225 0494 2

Printed and bound in Great Britain by
Richard Clay (The Chaucer Press) Ltd.,
Bungay, Suffolk.

CONTENTS

CHAPTER ONE

WHAT IS HYPERTENSION?

Briefly, hypertension is the medical term for high blood-pressure. For the whole span of our life we have to live with our blood-pressure, for it represents the force that must be exerted by the heart in order to propel the blood-stream through the arteries and onward through the vast network of the smaller blood vessels and the much smaller capillaries by which blood is conveyed to every part of the body.

Normally we are quite unaware of this continuous, forceful process of the blood circulation. Moreover, when some degree of abnormality of the blood-pressure does develop the person concerned may be totally unaware that any such state exists, and possibly would never know unless, for one reason or another, a measurement of the blood-pressure is carried out. Thus, if and when such a measurement is taken, and found to be 'too high', a sense of surprise or even positive fear is often created in the mind of the person concerned and this may, in some cases, become an obsession.

Fear and Anxiety

In view of the frequent development of overtones of fear and anxiety associated with the idea of hypertension, a brief description of the circulatory system may serve to explain the factors involved.

The heart is a hollow organ mainly composed of a special form of muscle termed cardiac muscle which continuously contracts and relaxes rhythmically, pumping the blood by means of each contraction (heart beat). The heart is, in fact, a double pump. As the heart contracts the blood in the left side (the left ventricle) is forced past a valve into the largest artery, known as the aorta. The aorta also has muscular walls and, in health, is strong and elastic. With the heart beat the powerful surge of blood distends the aorta which at once recoils and closes the aortic valve, thus preventing the blood flowing back into the heart.

Thus the blood is propelled from the aorta to the arteries (which themselves have elastic muscular walls) and beyond to the smaller arteries and so to the arterioles, which are smaller still, and so onward through the vast network of the capiliary beds which are situated in all parts of the body. It is estimated that there are about forty thousand million capillaries in the average adult body. Only about one quarter of these are opened at one time when resting, the remainder progressively opening up with increasing exertion.

Primary Duties of Circulation

As the blood passes through this network of small vessels it performs its primary duties, namely absorbing the products of digestion from the intestine and conveying these first to the liver, the body's chemical factory, for processing and thence to the living cells via the blood and tissue fluid (which itself is formed from the blood-plasma).

In these processes of digestion and assimilation the nutrients are prepared for assimilation by the cells, with large molecules being broken down to small ones (e.g. large protein molecules broken down to their small units known as amino acids), which are then enabled to pass through the enveloping membranes of the cells for the purposes of growth, maintenance and repair of tissues. This building-up process is termed anabolism.

Simultaneously, the waste products, mainly broken down protein and the gas, carbon dioxide, which is the product of oxidation processes, all pass out of the cells through the cell membrane into the tissue fluid to be transported into the blood-stream and so to be excreted, mainly by filtering through the kidneys. There is also some excretion through the skin and gaseous wastes pass out through the lungs.

Metabolic Processes

The processes of breaking down and excreting of tissue

wastes are termed catabolism and are the other half of the total biochemical processes termed metabolism. These processes of anabolism and catabolism together ensure the cleansing and renewal of tissues. Their functioning is entirely dependent upon the blood circulation. Having passed from the arterial to the venous capillary beds and to the smallest venules the blood passes through progressively larger and larger veins and so to the great vein, the vena cava from which it passes to the right side of the heart. Here the second heart pump, the right ventricle, contracts to send the venous blood through the pulmonary artery into the lungs, where the blood discharges its gaseous wastes, mainly carbon dioxide, and recharges itself with oxygen from the air which we breathe.

The lung structures contain a very large number of tiny air sacs called alveoli (there are estimated to be about 750 million of these) which present an area to the air which we breathe. In fact, the total surface of the alveoli membranes if spread out have been estimated to be large enough to cover an area of about 1,000 square feet

Respiration

These figures emphasize the importance of the process of respiration by which the blood is purified continuously before it is once again passed to the left ventricle to be again pumped into the general circulation.

It may be readily understood that if in these circulatory processes the body's waste products are not efficiently eliminated they will cause the onset of self-poisoning (autotoxaemia) which in severe forms, as with kidney failure, may be fatal.

This brief description may enable the reader to visualize the importance of the role which the blood circulatory system has to perform, both in maintaining its mechanical functions and as a vehicle for the transport of sustenance to every living cell, and, conversely, as a means of clearing cell debris and other toxins and thus cleansing all the living tissues.

It should also be realized that hypertension is not in itself a disease. It is indeed a physical sign which is defined only by direct measurement. Taken into account with other factors it may be of considerable diagnostic value in assessing a person's state of health. There are numerous ways in which the heart may be called upon to maintain the unimpeded blood flow and in medical terms the possible causes of high blood-pressure are multifactorial.

No Direct Symptoms

There are no symptoms which are directly and consistently indicative of hypertension. Thus many persons suffering from headaches or giddiness (vertigo), head noises, shortness of breath, fatigue, palpitations, insomnia, or any combination of these may come to the conclusion that they are due to high blood-pressure, though each and every one of these may be due to quite different causes. Although by feeling the pulse a qualified practitioner may conclude that a patient has a case of hypertension, only by actual measurement, using the instrument with the peculiar sounding name of the sphygmomanometer, is it possible to determine the blood pressure with any degree of accuracy.

The sphygmomanometer is an instrument which works on the same familiar principle as the barometer: pressure is measured by balancing against a column of mercury in a tube. A water barometer would require a head of over thirty feet high but as mercury is 13 per cent times as heavy as water the normal atmospheric pressure will balance 760 millimetres of mercury. There are now also sphygmomanometers which work on the aneroid principle of measuring atmospheric pressure.

Measuring Blood-Pressure

Most people are familiar with the cuff which in measuring blood-pressure is wound around the upper arm and inflated while the operator listens for the pulse through the stethoscope. Immediately the pressure in the instrument equals the pressure of the pulse beat and just beyond it, the pulse is no longer heard in the stethoscope and this point defines the highest point of pressure exerted by the heartbeat. This is known as the systolic pressure.

As the pressure in the cuff is gradually reduced by releasing a valve the column of mercury steadily falls until it comes to a point where the beat is no longer heard. At this point the reading of the height of the mercury gives the diastolic pressure, which is the residual pressure between heartbeats where for an instant the heart is resting. The diastolic pressure relates to the recoil of the elastic muscular walls of the arteries.

The difference between the systolic and the diastolic pressure is termed the pulse pressure. Until comparatively recently the diastolic pressure did not receive much attention but in recent years more importance has been accorded to this lower figure maintained during the brief resting interval between beats of the heart.

'Normal' Blood-Pressure

It will be asked, what is normal blood-pressure? Firstly, the answer is that it is not a static figure – in fact it can vary from day to day and even from one moment to another. This statement calls for some further explanation. When speaking of a normal blood-pressure not merely a single figure is to be considered but a range of pressures must be visualized which may vary according to our state of activity at the time and a number of other variable factors, as will be further explained.

Up to recent years the criterion was accepted as being approximately 100 plus the age of the individual (the figures are expressed in millimetres of mercury), so that the normal at age 20 would be 120 and at age 70 normal would be considered to be 170, etc. More recently blood-pressure readings above 150 to 160 systolic and 90 to 100 diastolic are the figures above which, if persistent, a person is said to be suffering from essential hypertension.

It is, however, admitted that when the effect of age is taken into account there is no sharp dividing line between normal and hypertensive blood-pressures. The above figures represent the pressure in the large arteries as the arterial blood leaves the heart. As the blood circulates through the system the blood-pressure declines as it approaches the capillaries. At the point where the right heart pump, the right ventricle, discharges the venous blood into the pulmonary artery to enter the lungs the pressure will be about 15 to 16mm systolic and 7mm diastolic.

With these few facts in mind it will be easier to consider the significance of hypertension and its possible causes, enabling the individual or the doctor to choose a treatment which may be both effective and lasting.

CHAPTER TWO

WHAT DETERMINES OUR BLOOD-PRESSURE?

In the preceding chapter the circulatory system and its vital mechanical processes by which the blood circulates, and upon which our continued survival depends, have been briefly described. From this it is possible to gain some understanding of the factors which may affect the blood-pressure, so that it may be said to be too high and thus that the person concerned is suffering from hypertension.

Although, as already mentioned, hypertension is not in itself a disease, the use of this specific medical term may imply to many people that it is in itself an entity. This is in accordance with the usual medical practice of giving to each manifestation of symptoms a specific name and hoping to prescribe in each case a specific remedy, for which the doctor looks to the drug manufacturers to supply. Such reliance on drugs for treating hypertension is far from being satisfactory, as will be explained.

A Direct Measurement

The systolic blood-pressure is, of course, a direct measurement of the force of the heart beat which is necessary to overcome the resistance offered by the system of blood vessels and is a load which the heart must continuously carry, though it is a task for which it is admirably competent in normal health. In fact the superb efficiency of the heart is truly wonderful. This little pump with its action cycle repeated about 100,000 times a day weighs only about 9 to 12 ounces in the adult, yet it may be expected to work continuously for 70 years or more with little or no particular attention or servicing as is necessary with man-made pumps. In some cases it is still functioning after 90 or 100 years and there are even rare exceptions of a few persons still living at the age of 130 or more.

It must be asked, however, why, in view of the heart's tough efficiency, there is now throughout the most highly civilized modern industrial societies a higher incidence of cardiovascular disease allied with hypertension than ever before, in spite of vast expenditure on medical services. (The costs of the National Health Service for 1976 were stated to exceed £6,000 millions, in spite of drastic cuts.) Any reduction of this modern scourge must by nature depend first on getting to understand the causes of this situation. A few further facts may be helpful in this respect.

When the resting pressure persistently exceeds the arbitrary figures of 150-60 systolic and 90-100 diastolic it is said to be *benign essential hypertension,* perhaps even up to readings as high as 200 to 210 systolic and about 110 diastolic. But higher than this, with such readings as 260 systolic and 150 diastolic, is regarded as being *malignant hypertension.* These again are arbitrary figures but blood-pressure of this order must be regarded as a danger signal and from the point of view of life insurance would be considered a poor risk. In all these conditions the strength and resilience of heart muscle and vascular walls are determining factors.

Maintenance of Efficiency

There are two main factors which enable the heart to maintain its remarkable continuous efficiency. First and foremost, the heart muscle is a special type of muscle which is not found in any other part of the body and is also served with a very highly developed system of blood circulation directly supplied by two arteries, the right and left coronary arteries, which are strategically situated at the entry to the great artery, the aorta, thus ensuring that the heart has first call on a liberal supply of the purified and oxygenated arterial blood as it leaves the left ventricle into the general circulation. This ensures that the blood flow with its nutrients to supply the cardiac muscles is about ten times more than to the other organs and tissues of the body.

Secondly, it may be wondered why the heart, working so continously, does not normally fail from fatigue. This is because the heart relies for its much-needed rest on the brief period (about half a second) in the phase of diastole between beats which is normally sufficient to maintain the cardiac process in balance. Furthermore, unlike any other organ or body tissue, the greatest flow of blood takes place during the period of diastole.

The Heart's Functional Efficiency

A brief comment on the functional efficiency of the heart was expressed by A. Rendle Short, M.D., F.R.C.S., Professor of Surgery, University of Bristol, in his book *Wonderfully Made* (Paternoster Press, 1953) as follows: 'It [the heart] performs the astonishing function of contracting down on the contained blood 60 to 70 times a minute, night and day, year in and year out, throughout our whole lifetime, and except for a few unfortunates, so quietly and comfortably that we never give it a thought. So long as its blood supply is maintained, it is proof against fatigue, in spite of its immense exertions.'

Unfortunately, the few unfortunates of that time have subsequently increased up to the present time when diseases of the circulatory system (cardiovascular and cerebrovascular diseases) comprise one half of all deaths. Obviously, such a major problem has excited much speculation concerning the possible causes of these diseases, of which hypertension is a presenting symptom.

The Psychiatric Viewpoint

From the psychiatric point of view nervous tension or anxiety neuroses have been seen as largely responsible for this situation and doses of 'tranquillizers' have been and still are prescribed. Anti-hypertension drugs are given, not to treat the causes of hypertension, but to act on the nervous system so as to block the nerve impulses which control the tone of the muscular structures of heart and blood vessels. Such drug treatments are no more than temporary expedients, acting in each case only about as long as the time for the next dose and in every case accompanied to a greater or lesser extent by side effects, most of which are detrimental to health and frequently dangerous, while none are likely to restore the patient to a true state of health.

Some Dawning Light

However, some light has recently dawned upon some sections of medical thought from unexpected sources. The existence of comparatively rare cases of longevity, hitherto generally disregarded, have attracted more attention. The point is that the best examples of superb health and active longevity are found, not in the centres of urban civilization with their programmes of care and social welfare allied to much doctoring, but are almost exclusively found among the few remaining primitive, isolated communities still living in their traditional environment and with their traditional dietary of whole, unprocessed foods.

The existence of such examples of positive natural health, persisting even in old age, has been observed and recorded first mainly by individual observers. When Robert McCarrison (later Sir Robert McCarrison) was appointed surgeon to the Gilgit Agency in the Himalayas over a period of seven years (1904 to 1911) he was profoundly impressed by the inhabitants of the State of Hunza, a community living in an isolated mountain valley in that region of Northern India. There he found a people characterized by superb fitness and health and active longevity with freedom from all manner of diseases. McCarrison carried out extensive researches all of which emphasized the supreme role of dietary to account for the Hunzas' excellent health even in old age. His findings were published in his book *Nutrition and Health.*

Other Primitive Communities

A further example of great significance to our present health situation was provided by Dr Weston Price, a member of the Research Commission of the American Dental Association. Dr Price carried out a world-wide series of field studies over the years 1931 to 1936, travelling from Greenland to New Zealand, visiting all five continents, to investigate the habits of primitive communities among whom dental decay and malformed teeth were virtually unknown. Fortunately Dr Price's researches opened a wider field of knowledge for he was able to relate these native diets not only to dental excellence but also as determining a high level of health and freedom from the chronic degenerative diseases of industrial civilization. Dr Price found that mortality levels from cardiovascular diseases were to be found only in certain areas in proportion to the length of time they had been exposed to the effects of modern civilization with its sophisticated foods.

Dr Price's findings were published in his book *Nutrition and Physical Degeneration* (published by the American Academy of Applied Nutrition, Los Angeles, 1939). Much more information to the same effect has followed the researches of Sir Robert McCarrison and Dr Weston Price. Similar facts and conditions have been verified and well documented concerning the health and longevity of relatively isolated communities in the Caucasus region of the Soviet Republic of Georgia.

Further Examples

Again, in Samson Wright's textbook of *Applied Physiology* (12th edition, 1971) it is stated that 'South Sea Islanders show little, if any increase in their mean blood-pressure level with age' but 'would-be inhabitants of developing townships show a remarkably increased tendency to hypertension.'

Once again, Dr David Davies reported concerning the inhabitants of a community in the Andean region of Vilcabamba in Equador (*New Scientist,* 1 February 1973). These people are found to be in excellent health with cardiovascular disease and hypertension being almost non-existent. An unusually large proportion of these people are centenarians, the oldest inhabitant being a certain José David whose birth was authentically recorded in 1840. Living actively to ages of 110 and 120 is not uncommonly rare. The majority of these people are vegetarians.

Other observers investigating primitive tribes in Africa have again found evidence of freedom from cardiovascular troubles with hypertension while living their traditional way of life including their native foods. Surgeon Captain T. L. Cleave, M.R.C.P. in his book *The Saccharine Disease* states concerning hypertension: 'among primitive peoples on a very simple natural diet these conditions are rare'.

Our Industrial Situation

In comparing the present situation in our industrial civilization, where hypertension and its associated cardiovascular diseases and coronary thrombosis are becoming more common even in the younger people, while a large proportion of our older people, far from being generally fit and enjoying active and useful lives are too frequently existing in a state of 'medicated survival' with failing powers due to premature senile degeneration, we might well imagine that between them and those primitive people described above there was some impassable hereditary barrier condemning us to suffer these degenerative conditions.

There is, however, strong evidence against such a negative conclusion. This evidence is that when members of these primitive communities leave their natural environment to live and work in modern industrial urban civilization and *adopting our dietary habits* then within a comparatively short time they begin to suffer from our civilized diseases almost all of which were virtually completely unknown to their ancestors in their natural environment.

The Dietary Key

It should be particularly noted that in all the above field studies concerning primitive peoples the paramount importance of their dietary of traditional whole foods was fully recognized and recorded by each and every investigator concerned.

Further evidence from numerous sources is progressively being accumulated in support of the view that modern 'civilized' diet is the major factor in causing hypertension and its associated cardiovascular diseases. Obviously some changes in our nutritional habits are urgently needed, both to prevent the onset of these degenerative changes and also to materially relieve and improve the condition in those whose blood-pressure is already a danger signal. In many cases this may add years of life expectation with increased vitality and in many cases will not only halt further degenerative changes but may also achieve positive improvement in the cardiovascular system with a correspondingly improved standard of health.

To achieve such desirable aims this book is intended to provide necessary helpful guidance in simple terms.

CHAPTER THREE

CAUSES AND CURE

Many of our vital processes are remarkable for their constancy and stability under varying states of activity and changing environmental factors, For example, the body seldom varies more than a few degrees from the normal 98.4°F (37°C) and the alkalinity of the blood is controlled to remain very close to the normal figure of pH 7.4 and so forth. With the blood-pressure, however, quite considerable variations are normal in accordance with circumstances, rising and falling according to our immediate state of rest or activity.

Thus in vigorous exertion the heartbeat strengthens and its rate increases in proportion, thus necessarily increasing the blood-pressure, all of which should soon return to normal on relaxing the effort. Similar rises in blood-pressure may result from emotional stress or nervous tension, These effects are perfectly natural unless over-exaggerated and prolonged.

Nature's Balance: Homeostasis

For the control of these variable factors within normal limits, known as homeostasis, there is an elaborate mechanism provided and controlled by a special section of the nervous system known as the autonomic (meaning self-governing) system which works in conjunction with the endocrine glands which secrete hormones (sometimes referred to as the chemical messengers). The autonomic nervous system is subdivided into two parts known as the sympathetic and the parasympathetic system respectively. This 'self-working' nervous and endocrine system largely controls all these mechanisms of the body over which we generally have no conscious control and which if we had to control we should find life to be quite impossible. Imagine what it would be like to have to supervise all our digestive processes, plus remembering to breathe continuously and simultaneously operate a large number of other vital functions, including our heart speed and strength of beat, in addition to controlling our blood-pressure to meet all circumstances.

In all these activities the autonomic nervous system normally serves us very well indeed. The sympathetic division of these nerves prepares us for physical activity, the so-called 'fight or flight' situation, in which it is assisted by the hormone adrenaline. The heart beat quickens and strengthens, the blood circulates more rapidly, breathing quickens and deepens and the blood-pressure rises to meet the circumstances. Simultaneously the processes of digestion and other 'vegetative' processes slow down or stop.

As soon as the phase of activity ceases with the crisis being over the parasympathetic nervous system takes over so that the heart rate, breath rate and blood pressure return towards their resting level and digestive and other vegetative processes resume their usual activity.

Margins of Safety

In such varying circumstances if the heart and blood vessels are healthy and efficient the stress involved is easily tolerated with good margins of safety. If, on the contrary, there is any abnormal resistance to the blood circulation the blood-pressure will be proportionately forced to operate over a higher range of pressure, both systolic and diastolic, in all states of activity, stress and even while at rest. In Chapter Two it has been indicated that under natural circumstances these processes and their associated structures are self-servicing, maintaining their functions possibly for nine, ten or more decades while nowadays they are breaking down in an alarming number of cases in the third decade of life and onward. There is therefore a pressing need to gain greater understanding of the underlying causes of hypertension and their relationship to the associated diseases of heart and blood vessels, and from this knowledge to decide what should be the basis of treatment.

Moreover, with those whose blood-pressure remains

normal the same principles and practices will apply in order to keep it normal, on the old but wise adage that 'prevention is better than cure'.

Adaption and Maladaption

Firstly, in order to accommodate to the usual variations of blood-pressure as described above, the normal controls are more than adequate, enabling the blood-pressure to adapt so as to meet all the ordinary and many of the extraordinary variations of stress and activity which may be encountered. It is only when maladaption develops that hypertension follows. We have to remember that the most prevalent diseases in modern civilized communities are the chronic degenerative diseases. Thus when hypertension develops, the primary causes of maladaption are subsequent to degenerative changes in the blood vessels in which the walls of the arteries may lose their texture, strength and elasticity with the development of arteriosclerosis (hardening of the arteries) or atherosclerosis (with formation of fatty deposits on the inner walls of the arteries).

In many cases there is also what is named renal hypertension in which there is a degree of loss of kidney function following degenerative changes in these latter vital organs, usually with progressive deterioration or destruction of the microscopically small kidney filtering units, the nephrons. Thus a number of factors combine to cause degenerative changes in vital organs, particularly the kidneys and the cardiovascular system.

Harmful Food Factors

First and foremost there are harmful factors in modern food which, after digestion, pass into the blood-stream through the walls of the intestine. If the diet is badly balanced, with some food factors in excess and deficiency in others, this may cause a relative acidosis and in many cases will result in excess weight (obesity) problems. Such nutritional defects also may result in faulty elimination of the products of catabolism (see page 9) leading to retention of toxic tissue wastes, mainly through kidney weakness.

Moreover the modern processes of refining foods frequently change a whole, nutritious food into a potentially dangerous one. Over and above these factors there are the thousands of chemicals used in today's commercial food processing and in farming and gardening, any or all of which we may imbibe and absorb from the popular foods of modern times.

Iatrogenic Diseases

With these foreign substances must be included the majority of modern drugs, many of their 'side effects' being, in fact, medically-induced diseases (the so-called 'iatrogenic', meaning doctor-induced, diseases.)

Thus with increasing weakness and damage to blood vessels the efficiency of the circulation will be affected and there will also be changes in the blood itself, increasing viscosity and with a tendency to thrombosis, in addition to a rise in blood-pressure. In many cases this situation is responsible for causing coronary artery disease and possibly also strokes, both of which may attack suddenly those who have been presumed to be in good health. This is understandable if it is realized that whereas deterioration, damage or disease is visible in structures such as teeth, skin, eyes, throat, etc., and though the deterioration of veins may be apparent as varicose veins, haemorrhoids and the fragility of small veins and capillaries may often result in bruising, either spontaneously or with a very slight knock, most of the arteries lie deeper in the tissues than the veins so that degenerative changes are not apparent. Hypertension may be the only sign until the sudden blocking of a vessel or a haemorrhage occurs as in coronary thrombosis or stroke.

The Major Factor

Further evidence from numerous sources is progressively accumulating to confirm that modern civilized diet is the major factor in causing hypertension and its associated cardiovascular diseases. Obviously, some modification of our eating habits is urgently needed both to prevent the onset of these and other degenerative diseases and also to effectively treat, relieve and improve the condition in the very many people whose blood-pressure is already a danger signal. In many cases this may add years of life expectation with increased vitality, an improvement in the quality of life, which in many is now so much reduced, and the achieving of a positive improvement in a weakened cardiovascular system. The heart will be assisted to adapt to the reduced load and, moreover, there may result a degree of improved kidney function.

To achieve such desirable aims the following simple plan of self-help is intended to provide the necessary guidance in simple terms.

CHAPTER FOUR

GUIDELINES TO HEALTH

Many readers, including those suffering from hypertension, may be surprised and perhaps sceptical concerning the role of nutrition both as the cause and the remedy for this very common condition. 'Surely', they may say, 'if this is so the doctor would have told us.'

In answer to this there is conclusive evidence that the association between nutrition and health is not confined to isolated primitives as mentioned in Chapter Three. The laws of nutritional science are directly applicable today, as many persons have experienced under the guidance of qualified naturopaths or those relatively few doctors who practise on nature cure lines.

We Are What We Eat

Some 25 years ago two doctors in South London produced a book entitled *We Are What We Eat*. This book gave a detailed account of the results of a suitably modified diet of whole, natural foods planned under the doctors' guidance and observation in a Salvation Army Home for Girls in Sydenham, South London to replace the usual diet of the establishment. These girls were generally retarded in health, both physically and mentally. The results, as recorded by Drs A. B. Cunning and F. R. Innes, were greatly beneficial in terms of decrease of common illnesses and epidemics, improvement in physical condition and also, to the doctors' surprise, marked improvement in mental condition with a decrease in delinquency and general nervous tension and also with an improvement in their school work.

It might be expected that examples such as these would have influenced many doctors to apply these findings in their practice. Unfortunately, it appears that doctors, with few exceptions, hold a traditional objection to diet, regard their practice as being limited mainly to treating their patients 'as they are' and not in the main attempting to alter their patients' habits, especially their habits of eating and drinking. Thus patients may not generally expect more than a mention of some single factor of possible self-help, such as to reduce taking animal fats or, if overweight, to be told to reduce weight, though usually without adequate instructions as to how best this may be done safely and permanently.

The 'Wonder Drugs'

Also it may have been unfortunate for the progress of nutritional therapy that about the time of the Sydenham project these were also the earlier years of the 'wonder drugs', which caused much excitement in medical circles, creating the illusion of the 'breakthrough' of chemotherapy and inaugurating the era of synthetic drugs, as a result of which it was easy to imagine that in the not too distant future one disease after another would be 'stamped out', thus winning the 'war' against disease and heralding in a sort of medical millenium.

But instead of conquering disease this policy has led to the establishment, at enormous costs, of what has been termed 'the drug-dependent civilization', otherwise expressed as 'pills for everything'. As may well be expected, the vested interests of the drug manufacturers have not failed to encourage this trend with large sums spent in promoting their products to the doctors.

The Prescription Pad

The combined results of these pressures, plus the influence of medical training, greatly accentuated the use of the doctor's prescription pad. Thus, most frequently in cases of hypertension, in addition to anti-hypertensive drugs, prescribing is extended to include other drugs to treat symptoms, possibly including tranquillizers, sleeping tablets and diuretic drugs (the latter to force out through overworked kidneys excess fluid accumulated in the tissues largely as a side-effect of other drugs). Each of these drugs has its characteristic side-effects, resulting in the complications of iatrogenic disease. In a critical article concerning the scene of modern medicine Dr David Mendel, Consultant at St Thomas' Hospital, London, commented (*The Observer,* 18 December 1977): 'Medicine is not a very intellectual subject. Laymen and many doctors think of medicine as being largely a question of knowing enormous numbers of facts and fitting them in like the pieces of a jigsaw puzzle. Diagnosis is *a bit* like that – the really important decision is what to do with the patient when you have the diagnosis. If a patient has hypertension, but no symptoms, the extent to which the cause and treatment are pursued depends on the assessment of many incomensurable and uncertain factors. Here an entirely different factor enters the picture — *it's misleadingly called common sense, and it is a most uncommon gift'* (my italics).

It is *common sense* that we should relate the total intake into our body to our problems of health and disease. It is the primary factor determining the quality of our tissues and the way our body functions.

It is *common sense* to accept that in hypertension, as in many other forms of disease, diet is a principal cause or even in some cases the sole cause. Many thousands of sufferers who have turned to Nature Cure treatment, usually after unsatisfactory experience of other methods, and have personally proved its efficacy.

All too frequently the medical attitude with respect to diet, often at best a fragmentary one, tending to disregard the principle of *wholeness,* will tend to discourage the patient from embarking upon a course of natural treatment. The principle of *wholeness* recognises that with complex systems the whole is greater than the sum of the parts. This principle is easily appreciated in considering a purely mechanical analogy. Imagine all the parts of a car scattered over the workshop: separately they are meaningless. But skilfully assembled, entirely new properties appear. The parts become a whole to function as a motor car. If parts are missing or constituents are of poor quality function may be interfered with or may cease.

Haphazard Selection

The human body, far more complex than a car, is all too often expected to function efficiently however haphazard the selection of its components (nutrients from our food from the time of conception onward) may be. Some food factors may burden the body with excess, other important nutrients may either be omitted, or be in short supply, while deficiency foods and foreign substances (chemicals, drugs, etc.) may be part of the daily intake from the environment, either by choice or accident, the latter not so much supporting the living cells as insulting and damaging these vital components of the body.

We may well ask how does the body continue to function in view of such disruptive factors? That it does so often survive is explained by the fact that it possesses great powers of adaptation and compensation as well as its innate powers of healing and repair all of which enable the vital system to counteract and compensate in such ways as to enable life to continue even though capability may decrease as degenerative changes advance and the body progressively draws upon its reserves. For example, the system of endocrine glands with their hormone production, in health working so harmoniously as to be referred to as the 'endocrine orchestra', the harmonious balance of mineral salts, including trace elements (in all about twenty different salts), these and numerous other factors that maintain the balance of health may become progressively disturbed. Tne kidneys may suffer gradual loss of the filtration units, the nephrons, to the point where renal unsufficiency is in evidence and the body's toxic wastes are no longer efficiently excreted from the bloodstream. Hypertension may be one of the earliest signs of increasing stress.

Whole Natural Foods

The states of physical excellence of many primitive isolated communites are founded on dietaries of whole, unprocessed, natural foods, the traditional dietaries to which they and their ancestors have become adapted over many centuries. The present knowledge of nutritional science, which is an important part of the curriculum in the training of a qualified naturopath, enables us to understand something of the virtues of these primitive dietaries and also serves to reveal the faults and fallacies of the popular feeding habits of today and, what is more, to relate its errors to the majority of our civilized diseases.

Nutritional knowledge today, in common with the study of medicine, is to a considerable extent empirical and possibly will always be so. Unfortunately the knowledge is too often applied by orthodox nutritionists in a fragmentary manner with little regard for the principle of wholeness. To the chemist white sugar is merely a pure crystalline compound; the nutritionist, however, may regard it as a potentially dangerous, even destructive food, though sugar as incorporated in natural whole foods, fruit and vegetable, may be wholly beneficial.

Fibre and Roughage

Not many years ago bran, the outer portion of the wheat, was regarded as the refuse of grain, useless as food and because of its rough texture, harmful to the sensitive intestine. More recently it was found to be beneficial for the healthy functions of the colon which was found to need fibre for bulk and roughage. Now there are indications that the whole grain as in wholemeal bread (including the bran) may help to reduce the incidence of the form of sudden heart attack termed ischaemic heart disease (IHD) (*Medical News,* 30 March 1978).

Thus from being considered as no better than 'dirty white bread' in a few decades wholemeal bread appears as a life-saver – truly wholesome food. How the story has changed! It is thought that this newly-discovered virtue is related to the excellently balanced content of mineral salts in the whole grain, in particular iron, potassium and magnesium in 100 per cent stone ground wholemeal bread, in which the stone grinding prevents loss of bran and wheat germ.

This principle of wholeness must govern the planning of a diet for hypertension.

CHAPTER FIVE

NATURE'S WAY TO HEALTH AND HAPPINESS

While there are other possible contributory causes of hypertension these are secondary and, however important they may appear to be, are in some way related to or affected to the dietary factor, either directly or indirectly.

We cannot expect to safeguard our life and health unless we ensure that our transport system, the blood stream and tissue fluid circulation, is supplied with all the many natural nutrients to ensure the integrity of the many millions of living cells, to nourish, build up, repair and also to cleanse and remove our metabolic wastes which must be eliminated through the bowels, the skin, the lungs and, most of all, through the kidneys. On this our health and eventually our survival are totally dependent.

Nutritional Errors

While some of our popular foods may be wholesome and natural and such as the human race has been adapted to for countless generations there are many other items in our diet in which the nutritional errors, excesses and deficiencies have been grossly underestimated both by doctors and the general public. To many of the latter we have never been able to adapt, nor are we likely to do so because they contravene some of the basic laws of nature.

In *Medical News* (1 October 1975) Dr Malcolm Harrison reporting on a statement by Dr J. L. Richard, Chief of Cardiology at the National Institute of Health and Medical Research in Paris, said that, concerning obesity, 'weight loss through dieting is accompanied by a clear cut reduction in blood pressure', and he asked the question 'Is dieting the easiest way to control hypertension?' Dr Harrison left this question open without further answer or guidance.

The Failure of Drugs

If to some readers swallowing tablets daily might appear to be the easy way to deal with hypertension they may do well to consider the following objections:

(1) Drug treatment fails to remove the causes or to cure the condition. It merely temporarily 'blocks' the nerves controlling the muscles in the walls of the arteries.

(2) All these drugs are toxic and have both short- and long-term 'side effects' which may be severe. Long-term effects may damage vital organs, including the kidneys.

(3) Other drugs are frequently used to treat the side-effects of the first one. This may include diuretic drugs to counter 'waterlogging' (oedema), inorganic potassium to replace losses of this mineral, and in many cases also tranquillizers.

(4) Often the drug will eventually fail even to reduce blood-pressure. This effect, known as 'tolerance', will indicate a change of drug which in turn may again lead to further 'tolerance'.

Drug treatment cannot be said to restore health or to strengthen or renew weakened tissues but instead may result in degenerative changes, eventually leading to premature senility. Thus drug treatment may prove not to be the 'easy' or even the effective way, in recognizing which certain eminent doctors have even extolled the virtues of 'intelligent letting alone'. This, of course, would mean 'neglect' to those accustomed to being given pills for everything. This is why some such patients are given a blank tablet or pill known as a placebo.

Indeed, to do nothing to help the natural healing potential is not enough. Thus the answer to Dr Harrington's question is a positive 'Yes', providing that the sufferer will decide to adopt and persevere with the nutritional programme thoroughly and conscientiously. This will result, in the great majority of cases, in a marked, persistent lowering of blood-pressure, reduction of weight where necessary, while the gradual improvement of normal bodily functions, the removal of toxins and encumbrances, the strengthening of the heart muscles and blood vessels and the relief afforded to the kidneys and other organs will all contribute to an improving state of general health. Self-help in these and other ways may prove to be infinitely rewarding.

The Nature of Disease

The history of medicine may be very instructive. In earlier times dirt and poverty and periods of famine, bad housing and hygiene, bad sanitation and polluted water supplies produced the virulent fevers, smallpox, cholera, diphtheria and tuberculosis. These have virtually disappeared with the changes in the environment.

Now we have new hazards and the causes of death have changed. With modern transport the supermarket shelves are never empty. Most people now eat too much, many become obese and yet may suffer from the modern forms of malnutrition because many of the chemically processed edible preparations may be described as 'Foodless Food'. Chief among these products are the refined carbohydrates, namely white flour (widely used in bread, cakes, pastries, biscuits, etc.), white macaroni and white (polished) rice.

A further health hazard and a case for serious concern is also a refined carbohydrate, namely white sugar which is used in so many forms such as beverages – tea, coffee, cocoa, beer, and many soft drinks – and is also a main ingredient in ice cream, puddings, pies, cakes, biscuits, chocolates and sweets and in many other forms and products.

Anxiety Among Nutritionists

All these trends are causing anxiety and alarm among nutritionists and many doctors. The sufferer from high blood-pressure should be prepared to avoid such refined and overprocessed foods in favour of moderate amounts of the corresponding whole foods and cease to pander to his or her so-called 'sweet tooth'.

Before adopting the balanced wholefood plan for hypertension the following points should be noted:

(1) The plan differs in important ways from most of the numerous 'slimming' diets which are planned for rapid loss of weight and are often concerned mainly with cosmetic considerations. All too frequently these schemes are ill balanced, not intended as a

permanent habit of eating. The 'dieter' may feel unwell and most frequently these schemes are abandoned only for the weight to go up again. If 'slimming' pills are included in the scheme it may be still more dangerous and undesirable. Moreover, very many sufferers from hypertension are not obese and may in fact be underweight, but still in their case unsatisfactory dietary will have caused degenerative changes, possibly with hardened arteries, damage to kidneys, liver and other organs. Both fat and lean may be equally in need of a radical revision of their eating habits.

(2) Such temporary 'slim-quick' plans do nothing to cultivate and establish new and permanent habits of eating with which the obese shed their burden of superfluous encumbrance while the thin, perhaps equally badly-nourished person, after a small initial loss, will slowly but surely build strong and healthy tissue. Such a plan of dietary is sure to benefit all types of hypertensives, even with those whose blood-pressure still remains higher than average, because such a diet will serve to restore the strength and elasticity of the cardio-vascular structures.

CHAPTER SIX

CLEANSING AND RENEWING THE BLOOD AND TISSUES

Popular notions concerning nutrition are largely centred on carbohydrates, proteins and fats and to many people vitamins and minerals are 'something you get in plastic containers'. In reality the foods which are most essential to the human body are those natural whole foods that, in addition to the proteins, carbohydrates and fats, are rich in essential minerals and vitamins. These latter in respect of which very many people are comparatively starved; their natural but often neglected source is mainly in fresh raw fruits and vegetables in the form of raw salads.

These latter 'cleansing' foods, with their important nutrients are essential for a healthy bloodstream and no amount of vitamin and mineral tablets will compensate for an inadequate intake of the foods that are their natural medium.

The treatment for high blood-pressure if it is to be lasting and satisfactory should be as follows: commencing with a period of cleansing and eliminative foods, with two days of taking only ripe, raw fruits selected from grapes, melon, apples, pears, pineapple, peaches, apricots or cherries. From this list two kinds should be selected for each mealtime, giving priority to grapes and melon. No fluids may be taken during these days. Fruit skins must be well washed. If there is any dryness of the mouth between meals try slowly eating a few grapes.

It should be noted that the above fruits are the sub-acid type and that at this stage the more acidic citrus fruits should be omitted. This short period of fruit only diet is sometimes referred to as a 'fruit fast'. It is a means by which the digestive system may be rested and the body's metabolic and excretory powers appear to be relieved of their daily tasks of dealing with the usual food intake and are directed towards the catabolic processes of eliminating accumulations of toxic residues both in the circulatory system and elsewhere.

Thus, to follow the brief fruit fast, the next seven days of this initial period of special dietary should be continued as follows: days 1 to 4 as below, varying the juices, fruits and salad ingredients day by day.

On rising:	Half tumbler of pure, unsweetened fruit juice, selecting from grape, apple, or pineapple juice.

Breakfast: Fresh, raw fruit selecting from ripe apple, pear or melon.

Mid-morning: One cup of Barmene or Tastex alternating with Vecon.

Mid-day: A raw salad. Select any three of the following ingredients – shredded white-heart cabbage, watercress, parsley, onion and grated raw carrot.

With the salad a portion of cottage cheese or about 2 oz. (56g) of a white cheese such as Wensleydale or Caerphilly.

As a dressing to the salad natural yogurt may be used. If preferred the yogurt dressing may be flavoured with a little pure honey or with one or more of the following: chopped parsley, mint, finely grated onion, paprika or chopped chives.

Evening: Ripe raw fruit and natural yogurt. A cup of Barmene or Tastex before retiring.

Days 5 & 6: With salad add 1 medium-size jacket potato (eat whole, with skin).

Day 7: As 1 to 4 but add two slices 100 per cent stone ground wholemeal bread, lightly buttered.

The above nine-day plan of cleansing and renewal will have already resulted in a lowering of blood-pressure in a majority of cases. It will be observed that this initial part of the plan for treating hypertension consists mainly of raw food and this is for very good reasons which call for a brief explanation.

The Importance of Raw Foods

Just as animals in their natural habitat do not eat cooked foods so prehistoric man must have subsisted on raw food for centuries before learning to cook. It is significant that modern nutritional science has demonstrated that by means of heat treatment in cooking a number of valuable food factors are lost, damaged or destroyed in the process.

In contrast, civilized man has gone to the opposite extreme so that a conventional diet consists very largely of cooked foods. In fact there are many people who seldom, if ever eat any appreciable amounts of food that is not cooked or otherwise degraded by processing, which uses vast numbers of chemicals to colour, texturize, increase 'shelf life', restore tastes artifically, and so forth.

What is needed urgently in our present efforts to reduce the incidence of chronic disease is to restore the integrity and lost values of our basic foods. In this respect, to revert to a primitive diet of whole, unprocessed raw foods only may well be impracticable in our present life situation. It is, however, reasonable and practicable to ensure that a substantial proportion of our total intake of food consists of such natural foods in the form of fresh, ripe raw fruits and salads. Please note that cold cooked and diced vegetables, often included in conventional salads, are not to be included. All salad vegetables should be eaten raw, usually grated or sliced.

The Potential Danger of Salt

It is now generally known that salt should not be used either at table or in cooking in cases of hypertension. The whole food balanced dietary supplies the essential mineral salts in balanced proportions including sodium chloride (common salt) but the addition of salt disturbs the biological balance and it is now known to raise the blood-pressure and so worsen the condition. Added salt also retains unwanted fluid in the tissues and is also bad for the kidneys.

Recent medical reports on hypertension have included one from World Health Organization (W.H.O.) under the title *Eat Less Salt and Live Longer* (*The Observer*, 26 March 1978). A further report (*Medical News*, 16 February, 1978) advised that salt should be restricted in hypertension 'before resorting to drug treatment'. Baking powder, containing sodium bicarbonate should also be avoided.

Most people develop some sort of pattern in their eating habits. Some will take several meals per day plus frequent 'snacks' in between. At the opposite extreme are those who have one large meal per day, often when tired at the end of a day's work during which they may have had nothing more than a brief snack (usually starchy). The digestive system cannot be happy with either extreme. The balanced whole food plan as indicated below, in which one main meal is based on raw foods while the second main meal is based mainly on cooked foods, will ensure optimum supply of the many essential food factors while aiding digestion and providing interest and variety to the palate. The main meals may be interchanged as wished.

Further details concerning ingredients of salads and other recipes and helpful hints are given in Chapter Seven. These are indicated thus * by the appropriate meal.

As already stated, with our modern deficiency foods most people eat far too much, but if the nutritional value of the diet is right the emphasis should be on quality rather than on quantity and meals will be relatively light. Meals should be unhurried, a time of relaxation, physically and mentally. Food should be well masticated, remembering that the first stage of digestion is in the mouth. The evening meal should not normally be taken late. A well-balanced diet should contain about the following proportions: carbohydrate 20 per cent, protein 10 to 15 per cent, fats 5 per cent and fruits and vegetables 60 to 65 per cent.

The Balanced Wholefood Plan

First Day

On rising:	Small tumbler half each of unsweetened apple and carrot juice.
Breakfast:	Ripe, raw fruit. Choose from apple, pear, grapes, melon or other sub-acid fruits as available.
Mid-morning:	One teaspoonful yeast and vegetable extract (e.g. Barmene, Tastex or Vecon).

First Main Meal:	Raw salad with grated cheese and jacket potato, baked or boiled: eat whole including skin. Follow with fresh raw fruit and ½ pint (0.25 litre) of yogurt.
Tea:	1 cup of weak tea or dandelion coffee, no sugar.
Second Main Meal:	Slice of melon or a grapefruit (as starter). Follow with poached egg on green vegetable. Serving of cooked carrot (conservatively cooked).*

Second Day

On rising:	Fresh unsweetened fruit juice or vegetable juice.
Breakfast:	3 to 4 tablespoonsful of muesli with grated raw apple. Add a little milk to taste.
Mid-morning:	Cup of Barmene, Tastex or Vecon.
First Main Meal:	Raw salad with cottage cheese and 2 slices of wholemeal bread, thin spread of butter or vegetable margarine. Follow with vanilla or coffee or chocolate mould (obtainable from health food stores).
Tea:	Fruit juice or weak tea or dandelion coffee.
Second Main Meal:	Green vegetable and jacket potato, nutmeat rissole.* Follow with fresh fruit salad.

Third Day

On rising:	Pure fruit juice (choose from apple, grape or pineapple).
Breakfast:	Serving of prunes (soaked overnight) and served with 2 tablespoonsful of wheat germ. Follow with fresh fruit.
Mid-morning:	1 teaspoonful Vecon in hot water.
First Main Meal:	Salad with about 12 walnut halves. Two slices wholemeal bread or crispbread with thin spread of butter or soft vegetable margarine. Follow with fresh fruit.
Tea:	As before.

Second Main Meal: A serving of TVP (texturized vegetable protein) hotpot* with a green vegetable. Followed by stewed dates.

Fourth Day

On rising: Fruit and vegetable juice as before.
Breakfast: Fresh grapefruit, sweeten with 1 teaspoonful of honey or unsweetened.
Mid-morning: Weak tea or dandelion coffee (or fruit juice).
First Main Meal: Salad with 2 oz. (56g) cheese. 2 slices wholemeal bread, thin spread of butter or vegetable margarine. Follow with dried fruit, figs or apricots etc soaked overnight. Serve with 2 tablespoonsful wheat germ.
Tea: As before.
Second Main Meal: Cauliflower with cheese sauce. Whole jacket potato and green vegetable. Half pint (0.25 litre) of yogurt, flavour with a dessertspoonful of molasses or a teaspoonful of honey.

Fifth Day

On rising: Fruit juice or weak tea as before.
Breakfast: 3 tablespoonsful of muesli with grated carrot and apple or other fresh fruit. Moisten with milk.
Mid-morning: Yeast and vegetable extract as before.
First Main Meal: Salad with hard boiled egg. Follow with fresh raw fruit.
Tea: As before.
Second Main Meal: Green vegetable (generous serving) with a smaller serving of carrot or swede or onion. Portion of tinned nutmeat savoury (obtainable from health food stores).
Follow with baked apple, removing core from large cooking apple and stuffing with raisins or sultanas or dates and baking. If liked serve with agar-agar custard.

Sixth Day

On rising:	Fruit or vegetable juice or mixed as before.
Breakfast:	Dried fruit (choice of prunes, figs, apricots, etc.) – soaked in a little water overnight and served with 2 tablespoonsful of bran and one tablespoonful wheat germ. Add milk to taste.
First Main Meal:	Salad with raw mushrooms and chopped nuts. Jacket potato as before. Follow with fresh raw fruit.
Second Main Meal:	Runner beans and garden peas or other green vegetables in season. Carrots in a cheese sauce. Two slices of wholemeal bread with thin spread of butter or vegetable margarine.

Seventh Day

On rising:	Small tumbler of mixed apple and vegetable juice.
Breakfast:	Ripe raw fruit as in season.
First Main Meal:	Salad with 2 oz. (56g) of white cheese (Wensleydale, Caerphilly or white Stilton). Follow with fresh raw fruit salad and agar-agar custard.
Second Main Meal:	Green and root vegetable with mushrooms and poached egg. Follow with three tablespoonsful of muesli with grated raw carrot and apple.

This diet should be followed strictly for three to four weeks, following which the whole routine should be repeated.

While the above dietary includes dairy produce the flesh foods, meat, fish and poultry, etc., are not included. The advantage of such a well-balanced lacto-vegetarian diet has been repeatedly confirmed in naturopathic practice over many years, and also various medical publications have advised reduction of these foods, although comparatively little medical research in this matter has been published. But in 1971 a team of researchers from Harvard Medical School, headed by Dr Edward Kass, reported a study of blood-pressure in more than 300 people on a macrobiotic vegetarian diet. Their blood-pressures were found to be well below both local and national averages.

If possible it is desirable to obtain organically grown fruits and vegetables. Your local health food stores may know of local farms and market gardens which grow produce organically. If you have any sort of garden grow as much food as you can using your own made compost, rotted straw, peat, seaweed extract (or seaweed itself added to compost or mulched or dug in directly if near coast). Tomatoes may be grown indoors and sprouting seeds will greatly help used in salads, etc. Your health food stores may advise. An excellent leaflet on this is published by Thompson & Morgan, The Seedsmen, Ipswich, Suffolk.

CHAPTER SEVEN

SOME RECIPES AND HELPFUL HINTS

VEGETABLE JUICES

These are sold at health food stores. Otherwise juices of root vegetables (carrot, beet, swede, etc.). If no mechanical juicer is available it may be prepared freshly, after washing and removing blemishes, by grating finely on to a double piece of muslin, folding over and twisting.

MUESLI

May be prepared with 2 tablespoonsful of muesli base (sold by health food stores) with 1 tablespoonful of rolled oats. Soak overnight in 4 tablespoonsful of water. Next morning add 1 dessertspoonful of sultanas or raisins, 1 desertspoonful of nuts, whole or milled. Add grated raw apple and/or grated raw carrot. Alternately other fruits added as available.

SALADS

All raw root vegetables are delicious grated in salads with the exception of raw potato. Thinly-sliced raw leeks add flavour as also do chopped parsley, mint and other fresh herbs. White-heart cabbage has more vitamins than lettuce and so should be used, coarsely grated, mainly as a base. Raw red cabbage is also very pleasant and may be similarly used. Lettuce can be used once or twice a week to 'ring the changes'.

Grated raw turnip mixes well with a few added currants. Raw beetroot combines well mixed with natural yogurt. Grated swede may be combined with a few sultanas. The white-heart cabbage may be combined with fresh orange segments or with a few chopped dates – be adventuresome and experiment to your own tastes with the raw grated vegetables. As an example, make a base of thinly-shredded white-heart cabbage and two other grated root vegetables, to add colour include a sliced tomato or sliced cucumber (eat the skin) and chopped mint or parsley as decoration.

The permutations of the above raw vegetables are manifold, take your graters and see what you can do and surprise your friends with your many and varied salads. Remember that salads are as essential in winter as in summer using the grated vegetables in particular which, incidentally are much less expensive than summer salads out of season.

DRESSINGS

Corn oil or sunflower seed oil may be combined with lemon juice or cider vinegar as a dressing, adding a little honey if liked and a few fresh herbs to flavour.

Natural yogurt is excellent as a dressing, either alone or

mixing a third of a pint of yogurt with a small teaspoonful of honey. This can be flavoured with grated onion, chopped chives or parsley.

CONSERVATIVE COOKING

This method preserves flavour and minimizes loss of vitamins and should be done as follows: In minimum water (2 or 3 cupsful depending on size of saucepan and amount of vegetables) bring to boil and add vegetables cut or shredded (e.g. carrots in rounds or quarters, cabbage shredded, sprouts whole). Place lid on tightly, shake frequently to prevent burning, adding more water if necessary. All root vegetables can be cooked together. Time of cooking 10 to 20 minutes according to age and size of vegetables.

PROTEIN SAVOURIES

Rissoles

4 oz. (113g) packet rissole mixture (health food stores)
2 oz. (56g) grated carrot
2 oz. (56g) grated onions
Pinch of mixed herbs or chopped parsley

Place grated vegetables in saucepan with 1 cup of water. Simmer until nearly cooked, flavour with yeast extract to taste, add herbs and rissole mixture, mix well. Shape into 2 rissoles and place on greased baking sheet. Bake at 375°F (191°C/Gas Mark 5) for almost 30 minutes or deep fat fry (enough for 2 portions).

The following recipes are based on texturized vegetable protein (TVP) which in several varieties is now becoming widely used. These are generally very palatable and all are highly nutritious without any of the disadvantages of flesh foods (meat, poultry, fish, etc.). It is now being recognized that these foods are particularly beneficial to the cardio vascular system. Under the heading *Soybean steak for Healthy Hearts Medical News* stated: 'Substituting soybean textured vegetable protein (commonly referred to as TVP or textured vegetable protein in TV commercials) for animal fat protein produces a greater fall in plasma cholesterol levels than does a standard low lipid diet.'

Bolognese

4 oz. (113g) TVP mince
1 onion
1 carrot
2 tablespoonsful tomato *purée*
1 tablespoonful vegetable oil

Hydrate TVP according to directions on packet. Chop finely or grate onion and carrot. Cook the vegetables in pan with the oil and 2 tablespoonsful of water until half cooked; stir to stop burning. Add TVP and tomato *purée* and ½ pint (0.25 litre) of water. Simmer for 20 to 30 minutes. Serve with 100 per cent wholemeal spaghetti (2 to 3 portions).

Hot Pot

4 oz. (113g) TVP chunks
2 carrots
2 onions
3 sticks celery
1 parsnip
1lb (450g) potatoes, scrubbed and sliced with skin on
Yeast extract to flavour.

Hydrate TVP as directed on packet. Slice the vegetables. Place alternating layers in casserole of all ingredients, finishing with layer of potato. Heat enough water to cover all the ingredients, flavour with yeast extract to taste and pour into casserole.

Cook for 1½ to 2 hours until the vegetables are cooked at 350°F (177°C/Gas Mark 3) (2 to 3 portions).

Stew

4 oz. (113g) TVP chunks
1 large or 2 small onions
1 large or 2 small carrots
1 turnip or small swede
1 stick celery
3 tomatoes
Yeast extract to flavour

Hydrate TVP as directed on packet. Cut or dice vegetables and add to TVP in saucepan. Cover with hot water and simmer 20 minutes or until vegetables are cooked. Add yeast to taste and thicken slightly with wholemeal flour. The vegetables may be varied to taste and season (2 to 3 portions).

Cheese & Mushroom Quiche

½ lb 100 per cent wholemeal flour
4 oz. (113g) vegetable fat

Mix fat into flour until texture resembles breadcrumbs. Add water – this varies with the flour, usually 2–3 tablespoonsful, but more may be needed to make a fairly moist mixture. Roll out carefully on floured board. This amount will cover a 9 inch flan ring. For the filling:

3 oz. (85g) grated cheese
4 sliced mushrooms
2 eggs (beaten)
Scant ½ pint (275ml) milk

Cover the flan ring with the sliced mushrooms and grated cheese. Heat milk to near boiling (but *not* boiling) and pour into a bowl that holds the beaten eggs, tipping the egg and milk mixture backwards and forwards from basin to saucepan 2 or 3 times, then pour into flan case. Bake at 400°F (204°C/Gas Mark 5) 30 minutes or until cooked.

Variations on this recipe could be cheese and sliced

tomatoes, cheese and sliced onions, cheese and sweet corn (tinned or frozen) (6 portions).

AGAR-AGAR CUSTARD

1 pint fresh milk
2 teaspoonsful agar-agar
vanilla or almond essence
1 heaped dessertspoonful demerara sugar

This is for use with appropriate second courses in main meals. Mix the agar-agar with half a cupful of cold water until it is without lumps. Then gradually add the cold milk. Bring mixture to boil while stirring. Simmer for a minute. Serve hot.

Further recipes and advice providing variety and interest may be obtained from *'Everywoman's Whole Food Cook Book'* by V. & C. Quick (Thorsons Publishers Ltd).

Many people for occupational reasons have to take packed lunches. All too often this may constantly consist of white bread sandwiches. A little imagination will help to provide a much better light meal. Possibilities include: (1) A carton of yogurt followed by apples and cheese and, to finish, a few dates or figs. (2) A container of home-made cole-slaw with carrot, white-heart cabbage, etc., dressed with a little natural yogurt. Apple or pear or grapes to follow. (3) Hard-boiled egg, lettuce, watercress or celery in season. Follow with nuts and raisins.

The 'business lunch' is also a possible hazard. However, this has had so much publicity it is now usually possible to select from the menu or pre-arrange to have a suitable meal, e.g. fruit juice starter followed by a salad and finishing with melon or fruit salad. If you mention your reasons to your guest or host he should understand and it is even possible that he may be glad to join you in a not-so-heavy meal for the sake of his own health.

The Balanced Wholefood Plan in Chapter Six shows beverages to be taken between meals. It is generally better not to drink with meals and this diet, with fruits and vegetables and without added salt, will ordinarily provide ample fluid. Many people drink far too much fluid and thus tend to overwork the kidneys.

CHAPTER EIGHT

FURTHER BENEFITS AND REWARDS

With those who have been troubled with constipation the natural diet alone will banish this condition. Rare stubborn cases may take about 2 tablespoonsful of bran daily. A dessertspoonful of molasses is also helpful in such cases, at least until a more regular habit is established.

In many cases of toxaemia of pregnancy with hypertension the introduction of whole food vegetarian dietary has been found to be effective in reducing both the toxaemia and the hypertension to the benefit of the expectant mother and presumably to the baby.

Other Causes of Hypertension

Concerning other causes of hypertension, in virtually all of these the dietary factor is also involved directly or indirectly, often to an extent that serves to emphasize the primary role of nutrition.

Thus although lack of exercise is an important cause of high blood-pressure in so many cases the problem at first is not so much exercising to get fit as getting fit to exercise, a dilemma which may be resolved only by adherence to the dietary programme so that gentle exercise at first may soon be increased in stages as the benefit of the diet becomes evident.

Obesity

This sequence particularly applies to problems of reducing obesity which (contrary to the popular idea) is rarely, if ever, achieved by exercise alone and thus requires suitable dieting treatment for its success.

The nutritional advice herein given is planned to establish permanently improved health, which means that sooner or later we should, by following the plan, achieve our *weight for health.* Thus an underweight person, after a small initial loss due to tissue cleansing, will gain weight (however slowly) while on the same programme the obese person will gradually shed his or her encumbrance so that each should reach and stabilize at their weight for health, and what for them is the blood-pressure necessary for circulatory efficiency.

Again, the endocrine glands with their hormone secretions are frequently involved in weight problems. In many cases the diet will tend to harmonize the hormonal balance, but some cases have difficulty in controlling weight and special measures, possibly with longer periods of fasting, may be necessary. This should be undertaken only under the direction of a qualified practitioner. Those who are able to spend a period of treatment in a Nature Cure health hydro may thus obtain considerable benefit but must subsequently continue to observe the rules of diet in a common sense manner.

Nervous Tension

Another factor in hypertension may be self-imposed nervous tension, and states of anxiety, resentment and other negative emotional states may be added by the awareness of being a hypertensive sufferer, causing over-anxiety perhaps amounting to fear. As against this the knowledge that self-help by means of dietary and other methods is both available and effective and will itself tend to reduce stress and anxiety. Also some very helpful advice is available in the book *Relax Your Way to Health* by H. D. Cotton (Thorsons, 1974.)

Smoking

Among the hazards now well known to cause hypertension is smoking. This habit is not easy to give up but the generally increased sense of well being and renewed confidence engendered by following the plan herein advised should help to strengthen any resolve to give up or at least greatly reduce the smoking habit.

Independence of Drugs

Finally there is the matter of independence of anti-hypertensive and other drugs as prescribed in the orthodox treatment of high blood-pressure, with all their disadvantages described in an earlier chapter. However, as health improves and blood pressure eases as a result of the dietary and other natural treatments this will facilitate the reduction of dosage and eventual discontinuance of these drugs in which event your doctor should be pleased to support your decision. In any event, if a qualified naturopath and osteopath has been consulted he or she will advise how and when such withdrawal of drugs may be effected.

By following this dietary plan the majority of people with hypertension will achieve a lowering of blood-pressure with much benefit to their general health and well being.

Even in those cases where hypertension persists the diet may still be of inestimable help in assisting the natural powers of the body to achieve the maximum possible degree of adaptation under these adverse circumstances.